LLA
DW

10403238

TELEPEN

617.8
MAR

is due for ret   w.

D0715362

2000

Other Books in the Series

In Preparation

PATIENT HANDBOOK 24

Hearing Loss

Michael Martin OBE BSc
Head of Scientific and Technical Services,
The Royal National Institute for the Deaf

Brian Grover BTech MSc MIOA
Deputy Head of Scientific and Technical Services,
The Royal National Institute for the Deaf

Foreword by
The Rt. Hon. the Lord Chalfont
PC OBE MC FRSA
President of The Royal National Institute for the Deaf

CHURCHILL LIVINGSTONE
EDINBURGH LONDON MELBOURNE AND NEW YORK 1986

CHURCHILL LIVINGSTONE
Medical Division of Longman Group Limited

Distributed in the United States of America by Churchill
Livingstone Inc., 1560 Broadway, New York, N. Y. 10036, and
by associated companies, branches and representatives
throughout the world.

© Longman Group Limited 1986

All rights reserved. No part of this publication may be
reproduced, stored in a retrieval system, or transmitted in any
form or by any means, electronic, mechanical, photocopying,
recording or otherwise, without the prior permission of the
publishers (Churchill Livingstone, Robert Stevenson House,
1–3 Baxter's Place, Leith Walk, Edinburgh EH1 3AF).

First published 1986

ISBN 0-443-02802-8

Library of Congress Cataloging-in-Publication Data

Martin, Michael, OBE.
  Hearing loss.
  (Patient handbook; 24)
  Includes index.
  1. Deafness – Popular works. 2. Hearing disorders –
Popular works. 3. Hearing aids. I. Grover, Brian.
II. Title. III. Series: Churchill Livingstone patient
handbook; 24. [DNLM: 1. Deafness – popular works.
2. Hearing Aids – popular works. 3. Hearing Loss,
Partial – popular works.   WV 270 M382h]
RF290.M35 1986   617.8   86-2242

Produced by Longman Singapore Publishers Pte Ltd
Printed in Singapore

Foreword

Of every 10 people in this country, two suffer from some degree of hearing loss. This covers a wide spectrum, from those who experience minor difficulty in certain situations to the 100 000 or so who have no useful hearing at all. It is a problem of which the community as a whole is largely unaware, yet it means that literally millions of our fellow citizens have difficulty in using telephones or listening to the radio or the sound on television; they often cannot hear doorbells or alarm clocks and do not know when their baby cries. Most of them feel frightened and alone.

One of the most frustrating and depressing aspects of deafness to those who suffer from it is its invisibility. Most other disabilities are easily recognisable, but the deaf often seem to other people to be just inattentive or slow on the uptake. For this reason deaf people are often treated with less kindness and consideration than those who are blind or in some other way obviously disabled. At the same time, those who suffer from hearing loss are often reluctant to admit it and frequently try to conceal their condition rather than seek treatment or advice.

This problem is aggravated by the shortage of technical information expressed in the sort of language which makes it accessible to non-specialists. People suffering from hearing loss are therefore often quite unaware of what can be done to help them. Michael Martin and Brian Grover have performed an invaluable service in remedying this deficiency: *Hearing Loss* is written in an authoritative but clear and simple style which can easily be understood by readers with no technical or medical background.

After explaining the nature and causes of hearing loss (and, incidentally, discouraging the use of vague and often disparaging terms such as 'stone deaf' and 'deaf and dumb'), the authors deal with treatment and, in considerable detail, with the various hearing aids now available. There are useful sections on such associated subjects as tinnitus, lip-reading and auditory training.

Deaf people often claim that theirs is the loneliest disability of all, isolating them cruelly from the rest of the community, which often seems unaware of their condition or uncaring about it. For this reason it is important that this book should be read not only by those suffering from hearing loss and uncertain of what they should do about it, but by hearing people as well — especially those who are in frequent contact with the deaf.

1986   Lord Chalfont

Preface

This book has been written to answer in a straightforward way some of the questions that you may want to ask about hearing loss. Unfortunately, to many people hearing loss is still something to be hidden, not talked about, and this attitude is not helped by the general lack of non-technical information for those who want to find out about the subject. The more it is realised how much can be done to overcome the effects of hearing loss, the fewer will be the number of people who become isolated by it from their friends, families and others around them.

This book covers many aspects of hearing loss and will be of value to those who are just beginning to experience problems with their hearing as well as those with near total deafness. It should be of particular value, however, to the great number of people who, through advancing years, are facing increasing problems with their hearing and also those who have contact with people who must face the problem. It explains what can happen to the hearing system, what can be done to correct it, and gives practical advice on how to cope in various situations.

There seems to be much misunderstanding over the meaning of words and terms which are used to describe poor hearing. Some of these words will be explained, but, as our concern lies mainly with the practical problems faced by people with hearing loss, we have spent little time on trying to place people into categories. Consequently we have used the general term 'hearing loss' throughout much of the book to include all degrees of impaired hearing, however great or small these may be.

London, 1986   M. M., B. G.

Contents

1 What is hearing loss?

Is hearing loss common?

Recent surveys by the Medical Research Council's Institute of Hearing Research suggest that as many as 10 million people in the United Kingdom suffer some degree of hearing loss. Fortunately, most of these people have only a small degree of loss, which causes difficulty only in some situations. This book will explain what can happen to the hearing system and what can be done to correct it; it also gives practical advice on how to cope in various situations.

Like the other senses, hearing tends to deteriorate as we get older and, for this reason, we should not be too surprised to learn that the average age of people attending a hospital hearing aid clinic for the first time is about seventy. Nearly 2 million people in the UK either use or have used hearing aids and the stigma attached to wearing one is slowly fading. Chapters 4 and 5 deal with the different types of hearing aid, their uses and their limitations.

About 100,000 people have no useful hearing at all and, for them, even high-power hearing aids will probably be of little use. There are, however, other devices to help with particular problems. Some of these people will have been deaf since birth or early childhood and, while the numbers of children born with this handicap has fallen, at least one child in every thousand still has a serious hearing loss at birth.

How could it affect me?

If your hearing loss is not severe, you will probably have no problem talking face to face with someone who speaks clearly. However, when you are in a noisy environment or listening to someone at a distance you may have considerable difficulty. When listening to television or radio you may want to turn up the sound more than others would like and you may find that you no longer hear the doorbell or telephone every time it rings.

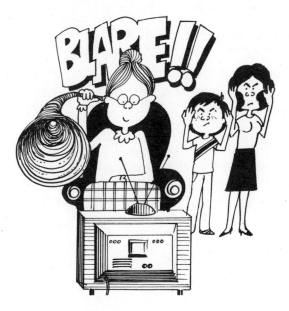

If your loss is more severe, you may have to rely on your lip-reading ability, even in face-to-face conversation. You may no longer be able to enjoy television, theatre and the cinema, and the telephone may become impossible to use without some form of assistance. Your work might be affected and you may even have to consider alternative employment. Nevertheless, there is nearly always something that can be done to minimise the problems you face. In fact, the most serious problem is doing nothing at all.

How does the ear work?

The ear is divided into three main parts, which are the outer, middle and inner ear (shown in Fig. 1).

The outer ear consists of the external part that we can see: the pinna and the ear canal. The purpose of the pinna is to collect sound, which is then passed down the ear canal to the ear drum. Near its entrance, the surface of the ear canal is covered with wax glands and small hairs to prevent the entry of dirt etc.

The middle ear consists of the ear drum, the ossicles (which are the three smallest bones in the body) and the cavity they bridge. The function of the middle ear is to pass the very small movements of the ear drum to the inner ear.

The inner ear is called the cochlea, which is a snail-shaped organ in which the vibrations received from the middle ear are turned into tiny electrical signals that pass along the auditory nerve to the brain.

Are there different types of hearing loss?

There are two main types of hearing loss. Conductive hearing loss leads to a loss of loudness which can be overcome by amplifying the sound and which can often be helped by medical or surgical means. Sensorineural (or perceptive) hearing loss, on the other hand, leads not only to a loss of loudness, but to a lack of clarity as well; in general, there are no medical or surgical means of help. This type of loss is sometimes, incorrectly, called nerve deafness. Unfortunately, in most cases of sensorineural hearing loss the lack of clarity cannot be completely corrected by

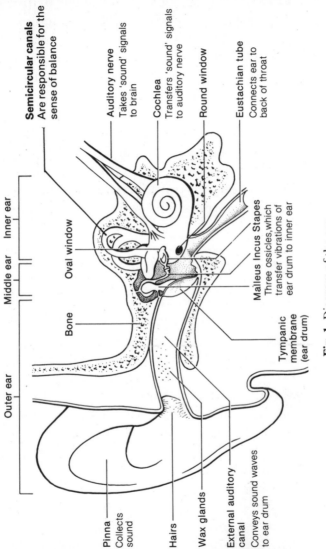

Semicircular canals
Are responsible for the sense of balance

Auditory nerve
Takes 'sound' signals to brain

Cochlea
Transfers 'sound' signals to auditory nerve

Round window

Eustachian tube
Connects ear to back of throat

Inner ear

Middle ear

Outer ear

Oval window

Bone

Malleus Incus Stapes
Three ossicles, which transfer vibrations of ear drum to inner ear

Tympanic membrane (ear drum)

Pinna
Collects sound

Hairs

Wax glands

External auditory canal
Conveys sound waves to ear drum

Fig. 1 Diagram of the ear

amplifying the sound. An appreciation of the difference between conductive and sensorineural hearing loss is vital to understand why some hearing-impaired people appear to be able to manage so much better than others.

The effect of conductive hearing loss is like trying to listen to someone who is speaking very quietly, or at a great distance. If the person speaks up or comes closer, you can hear and understand perfectly. Sensorineural hearing loss, however, will not only lead to a reduction in the level of sound (as in the case of conductive hearing loss), but it will also cause distortion, which means that, even when the sound is made loud enough to hear, it may still not be understood by the listener. The effect is a bit like listening to an unknown foreign language; you know that someone is speaking, but cannot understand what the person is saying. The outer and middle ear are associated with conductive hearing loss whereas the inner ear is associated with sensorineural hearing loss. As well as these, there are also some rarer forms of deafness.

If you have a hearing problem, you should

go to see your doctor. However, if you ever suffer a sudden, severe loss of hearing, you should go at once to the casualty department of your nearest hospital. With immediate treatment, your hearing might be restored.

How is hearing tested?

If you think you have a hearing loss, you should have a hearing test. There are good reasons for having this under medical

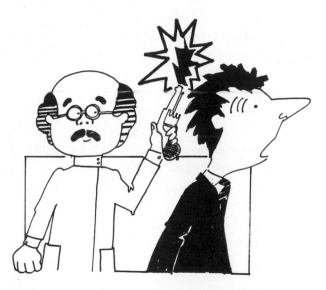

supervision, particularly if this is the first time your hearing has been tested. The result can suggest the cause of the hearing loss, the kind of problems you may face, and the treatment which should be tried.

Most hearing tests are given in out-patient clinics of local hospitals, the majority of people being referred by their family doctors. Although some rather complicated tests are used in special circumstances, a simple test of hearing ability, known as pure tone audiometry, takes only a few minutes. You listen to a series of tones, each of different pitch, which are presented as short bursts of sound, first to one ear and then the other. The loudness of each tone is reduced until you can just hear that it is still there. This point, known as your threshold of hearing, is marked on a chart called an audiogram (Fig. 2). Gradually a picture builds up of the range of sounds you can hear. Usually the tones are heard through headphones, but you may be fitted with a small vibrator, which goes behind the ear, to test for conductive hearing loss.

You may be given a test in which you listen

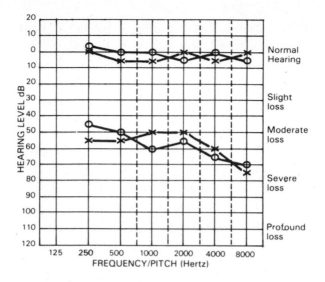

Fig. 2 A typical pure tone audiogram, showing the hearing of someone with normal hearing and someone with a hearing impairment. x = Left ear. o = Right ear

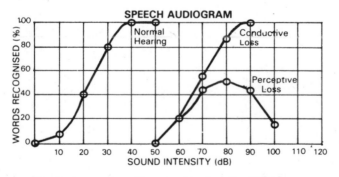

Fig. 3 A speech audiogram showing the difference between a person with normal hearing, a person with conductive hearing loss and a person with a perceptive loss. Note that a person with a perceptive loss may not understand all the words and making them louder may reduce understanding even further.

to lists of words or sentences which have to be repeated. This test can show the difficulty you may be having with conversation and is called speech audiometry. Figure 3 shows how the different types of hearing loss affect how well people understand speech.

How is hearing loss described?

It can be described either in words or numbers. We are probably all familiar with terms such as 'stone deaf', but these are not really very helpful in understanding a person's difficulties. Another term still occasionally used is 'deaf and dumb', but this is quite misleading, as most deaf people do have the power of speech, although they may be difficult to understand. These days this expression is generally felt to be socially unacceptable anyway. The problem is that people born with a severe loss of hearing find it extremely difficult to learn to speak normally. This is simply because other people's voices are not heard and therefore cannot be imitated. Moreover, they are unable to hear their own voices when they do try to speak.

The effect of different degrees of hearing loss

Decibels of hearing loss	Degree of impairment	Practical effect on hearing
Up to 25	Within normal range	Little effect
30–45	Mild	Difficulty with quiet voices
50–65	Moderate	Difficulty with many sounds
70–90	Severe	Cannot hear speech without a hearing aid
Over 95	Profound	Can hear only a little even with a powerful hearing aid

Scientifically, hearing loss (and sound in general) is measured in decibels (abbreviated to DB). An approximate relationship exists between the decibel hearing loss and the degree of difficulty it may cause (see the Table on page 12).

Sometimes people are given their hearing loss as a percentage, for example, 'You have a 50 per cent loss.' This may seem easier to understand, but it is not really a correct way to describe hearing; decibels should not be converted like this. One hundred decibels represents a very considerable loss of hearing, but it certainly does not mean total deafness, and it would definitely be worth persevering with a hearing aid in order to obtain some benefit.

For the purposes of compensation for hearing lost in a noisy place of work, a percentage 'disability' can be estimated; but, again, 100 per cent disability does not mean total deafness.

Is it rare to have noises in the head?

Unfortunately it is not. This condition,

known as tinnitus, is actually quite common and the noises may be heard in the head or else in one ear or both. Sometimes the person has a hearing problem as well, but often the hearing is quite normal. In fact nearly everyone experiences ringing in the ears at some time or another, often after exposure to loud noise.

There is no cure for tinnitus at the present time, nor is enough usually known to be able to say exactly where in the hearing system it is produced. However, a little device which looks rather like a hearing aid may help. It is called a masker, because the gentle rushing sound it makes may cover up or mask a much less pleasant noise in the head.

Some people find the noises almost unbearable..They are often worse at night before going to sleep and first thing in the morning. The most important thing is not to be alarmed. The noises are not usually a sign of a serious medical condition.

A small number of clinics specialise in the treatment of tinnitus; ask your doctor for information. If you want to know more about tinnitus or meet other people with the same condition, you can join the British Tinnitus Association, which will supply a list of self-help groups, run by people who share this problem.

Is there a connection between giddiness and hearing loss?

You can see from Fig. 1 that the inner ear connects with the semicircular canals, which help to provide our sense of balance. A condition can occur which results in loss of hearing, tinnitus and giddiness. This condition, known as Ménière's disease (after a famous French physician), can be very distressing and requires specialist treatment. Attacks may occur at intervals and the deafness and tinnitus may fluctuate. Sometimes the hearing will return to normal without any treatment.

Giddiness or loss of balance should always be taken seriously and you should seek your doctor's advice. There are many conditions which can lead to giddiness, some of which are connected with the hearing. You may well find, therefore, that if you suffer from this problem you are referred for treatment to an ear, nose and throat clinic.

Can hearing loss affect the voice?

This is only likely to happen if your hearing loss becomes severe. Most people with relatively minor loss can be reassured that their speech will remain normal. A more likely problem is that you may not be able to tell if you are talking too loudly or too softly. A hearing aid should alleviate this problem—which is another good reason for using one.

If a child is born deaf, or becomes severely deaf before learning to speak normally, it is very likely, however, that the quality of the voice will be affected. Such a person may be referred to as pre-lingually deaf.

2 What causes hearing loss?

Are there simple causes?

Wax is produced naturally in the outer ear canal and some people produce a great deal more wax than others. The simplest cause of hearing loss is a build-up of the wax in the ear canal; once this wax completely blocks the ear canal, you could have quite a noticeable loss of hearing. Fortunately, in most cases the wax is easily removed by a doctor or nurse. Something which has been pushed too far into the ear canal, such as a piece of cotton wool, can create the same effect; in fact you should never push anything into your ear, although some people do this in an attempt to clean the ear canal. The use of hair pins, matchsticks or cotton buds can lead to the wax being pushed beyond the point where it can leave the ear by natural means.

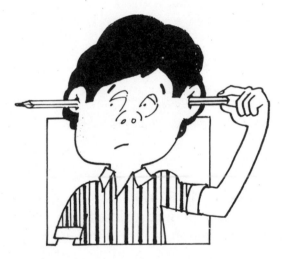

If you have a cold you may experience a slight hearing loss. This should disappear when you get over your cold. If you fly, or climb a mountain, you may experience a minor degree of hearing loss due to the difference in pressure between the air in the middle ear and the outside air. The problem will disappear if you blow your nose or swallow.

After being exposed to loud noise for a short while you may feel slightly deaf, but your hearing should slowly return to normal once you are out of the noisy environment. This phenomenon is called a 'temporary threshold shift'. Too much exposure to loud noise, however, could lead eventually to a permanent hearing loss. We will say more about this later in the chapter.

What are the common causes of hearing loss?

One common cause of middle ear (conductive) deafness is otosclerosis, a condition in which the little bones in the middle ear (the ossicles) get covered with a bony growth. This affects the stapes (the innermost bone) in particular. An operation called a stapedectomy may be undergone to overcome this problem (see page 29).

Infection in the middle ear can cause a build-up of fluid in the cavity, which may lead to temporary deafness and possibly a discharge from the ear. Perforations of the ear drum (which can be caused by blast) will also lead to conductive hearing loss.

Sensorineural hearing loss can be triggered by a wide range of viral infections such as mumps and measles. Other causes of this type of hearing loss include use of certain drugs and exposure to noise. As we become older a loss of this kind is quite normal.

Do earaches matter?

Earaches matter because they are a sign that something is wrong. They can be caused by such things as middle ear infections and bad teeth. If the earache persists, see your doctor.

Is damage to the ear drum serious?

Many people think that if the ear drum is damaged you will become totally deaf. This is quite untrue. However, damage in the form of a perforation or even a rupture of the drum will cause some hearing loss of the conductive type. If the eardrum does not heal naturally, surgery can sometimes effect a repair. Surgeons sometimes deliberately make holes in the ear drums of children who have a build-up of fluid in the middle ear. This small operation, where a grommet is inserted to prevent the ear drum from closing, provides ventilation of the middle ear and allows the thick fluid, often called 'glue', to disperse.

If you have a perforation of the ear drum and you want to go swimming, earplugs must be used to prevent water from entering the middle ear.

Why are some children born deaf?

If a mother-to-be contracts rubella (German measles) in her third month of pregnancy, there is a risk of the baby being born with one or more serious disabilities, one of which is deafness. This is why doctors strongly recommend that girls should be immunised against the disease.

A difficult birth, particularly when the

baby gets insufficient oxygen, can cause deafness. Hereditary or genetic factors are also very important; in some families deafness passes from one generation to the next. Genetic counselling by a specialist with knowledge of deafness is very important and can reveal the chances of deafness being transmitted in this way.

Many young children who are born with normal hearing suffer from middle ear problems, often between the ages of three and ten years old. These problems may lead to only small and temporary losses of hearing, but they can cause a child's education to fall behind if they are not treated promptly.

Can drugs damage hearing?

Unfortunately, a number of drugs are ototoxic, which means that they are capable of damaging the hearing system. Some of these are powerful life-saving drugs, but others are widely used remedies. Even aspirin, taken in large quantities, can affect your hearing. Some drugs produce tinnitus, so if you are taking medicine that seems to produce dullness in your hearing, or noises in your head, tell your doctor. With some drugs the loss is only temporary, but with others it could be permanent.

Why do older people go deaf?

As we grow older our bodies slow down. Our hearing, just like our sight, may become impaired, but, whereas people will seek advice about sight problems, they are often very reluctant to do anything about their hearing.

Hearing loss in old age has a medical name: presbyacusis. This is the perceptive type described in Chapter 1 and it is due to changes in the inner ear (and to some extent in the nerve which leads to the brain). Usually the loss is gradual; it affects nearly everyone, although some people suffer more than others. High-pitched sounds are always the first to become difficult to hear, making it hard to catch certain words. Quite often the person is not aware of this and blames others for mumbling. In fact it is often only after prompting from the family or friends that the person considers getting a hearing test, and then possibly a hearing aid. It is important for people to face up to the fact that they have problems with their hearing as soon as possible. Unfortunately too many people persevere for many years with hearing which is becoming worse and are quite elderly before they are prepared to ask for help.

Can noise damage my hearing?

Boilermaker's ear and Weaver's deafness are just two names which remind us of how work in noisy factories and industries has robbed many people of their hearing. So legislation is being introduced to limit the sound level in which a person may work without hearing protection. The limit will probably be set at ninety decibels; this is about equal to the sound inside an underground train. If the noise is any louder, the employer has to provide ear plugs or ear muffs for the workers. Even this level of noise is known to cause hearing loss in some people after a number of years of work. It is important to appreciate that it is not just the level of noise that matters, but also the amount of time you are subjected to it. The louder the noise, the shorter the time you should have to put up with it. Unfortunately some people are more susceptible than others to this sort of hearing damage, but it is not possible to find out whether you are one of these until it is too late. A good employer will ensure that the hearing of employees who are at risk is tested on a regular basis, in order to give advance warning of any impending problems.

There are many sounds which can damage your hearing; if you fire a rifle or use a chain saw, for instance, you should certainly wear muffs to protect your ears. You should also consider ear muffs if you need to use noisy do-it-yourself appliances (such as an electric drill) in a confined space.

Discothèques and rock music concerts are often thought to harm young people's hearing, but, while some bands definitely play too loud, most people do not go to such events sufficiently often to lead to a permanent loss of hearing. Nevertheless research is presently being undertaken to determine the degree of risk involved. The musicians themselves as well as staff who work in clubs and other music venues are probably at greater risk than the customers. A more recent worry is with personal stereo-cassette players, which can be worn for hours on end. As with any loud sound, hearing damage is a possibility when noise levels are too high, and common sense should prevail.If sensible volume settings are used, then potential problems can be avoided. It must be appreciated that it is the constant bombardment of the ear with loud noise which contributes to a possible hearing loss. It is also important to realise that such damage leads to a perceptive loss, which cannot be cured; moreover a hearing aid may give only limited help. Worse still, this loss is added to whatever loss you acquire as you grow older. So eventually loud music may contribute to hearing deterioration, even though it might not seem a problem at the time.

Can accidents cause hearing loss?

Accidents involving head injuries may cause deafness due to damage to the nerves that carry signals to the brain, or damage to the part of the brain that receives the auditory signals (called the auditory cortex). Blast may rupture the ear drum, and for divers there is a risk of damage to the ear due to large changes in pressure.

3 How is hearing loss treated?

What should I do about treatment?

If you ever suffer from a sudden severe loss of hearing, you should go at once to the casualty department of your nearest hospital. With immediate treatment your hearing might be restored.

Normally, however, you should first go to your own doctor. Your doctor can refer you to a specialist (usually an otologist) under the National Health Service for treatment at the nearest hospital's ear, nose and throat department, or can arrange for you to see an ENT consultant privately. Medical etiquette demands that you can only visit a consultant if referred by another medical person; this will normally be your own doctor. In some areas it is now possible for a GP to refer an elderly person directly to a hospital hearing aid department in order to avoid a potentially long delay in seeing a consultant. This is done on the assumption that the person does not require medical treatment, but, even so, if the staff in the hearing aid department are not satisfied in any way about the person's medical condition they will ensure that the person is referred back for appropriate treatment.

Can drugs help?

Drugs are used in the treatment of many problems concerned with the ear and hearing. In most cases the drugs are used to treat an infection or an underlying condition and, once this has cleared up, the drugs will be stopped. It is unlikely that drugs will be prescribed on a long-term basis. There are certainly no drugs that will cure a sensorineural hearing loss.

Will I need an operation?

Whether you need an operation or not will be decided by the otologist. However it is important to realise that different types of operations are undertaken and the majority of operations are done to correct problems in the middle ear.

Otosclerosis is a common condition in which a bony growth prevents movement of the ossicles (the three tiny middle ear bones), particularly the stapes. A stapedectomy operation replaces the stapes with a metal or plastic piston and has a good rate of success in restoring hearing to near normal.

Mastoid operations used to be quite common in the days when drugs were not available to treat infections of the middle ear, which could lead to an abcess forming in the mastoid bone. Fortunately, today mastoid operations are relatively rare.

Where the eardrum has a perforation, an operation called a tympanoplasty may be performed to close the hole. When successful, this operation can restore hearing almost to normal.

There are obviously a wide range of operations for specialised cases, but for the majority of people, the operations described above are those most likely to be performed. These are all done to relieve conditions which lead to conductive hearing loss. No operation can be performed to help the vast majority of people with sensorineural hearing loss.

What about a hearing aid?

For many people a hearing aid is going to be the only practical form of help.
This is particularly true for those with sensorineural loss, although it is often incorrectly said that hearing aids are of no use in such cases. Hearing aids can be obtained through the National Health Service or may be purchased privately (see Chapter 4).

Remember that using a hearing aid is really no different to wearing glasses, so do not be put off the idea of hearing aids because you think they make people appear older or somehow less active. Modern hearing aids are quite small and will help rather than interfere with your everyday activities.

4 Getting a hearing aid

Do I need a hearing aid?

Do you have trouble in hearing the door or telephone bell? Do you need the television louder than others would like? And do you find that other people always mumble? If so, you might benefit from a hearing aid. You should not worry that you might become dependent on it as a hearing aid should not affect your hearing loss (see page 51). It is far better to get an aid sooner rather than later when you may be struggling to hear; otherwise you may have already cut yourself off from people because it has become so difficult for them to communicate with you.

How do I get a hearing aid?

In this country there are two ways of acquiring a hearing aid. You can go through the NHS and get one from a standard range free of charge, or you can go privately to a hearing aid dispenser. It is important to realise that these two methods are completely distinct; there is no NHS assistance towards the purchase of private hearing aids.

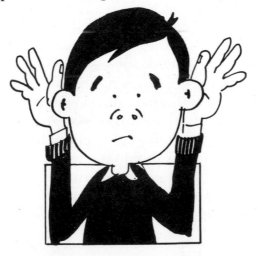

How do I get an aid from the NHS?

To obtain a hearing aid through the NHS, you first have to go to your doctor. If your doctor thinks it necessary, you will be sent as an out-patient to the nearest ear, nose and throat department of a hospital. At the hospital a medical consultant will examine your ears and may arrange for a hearing test (as described in Chapter 1). The consultant will then decide whether you need a hearing aid, or whether some other form of treatment may help you. If a hearing aid is recommended, you will be sent on to the hearing aid department. An aid will then be selected for you and an impression taken of your ear with silicone rubber as a first step in the preparation of an individual earmould (the part that goes into your ear). Some time later you will have to return to the hospital to be fitted with your hearing aid and to be shown how to use it. There is no charge for the hearing aid, or replacement batteries, or any future service.

The time taken to obtain a hearing aid may vary from just a few weeks to as much as two years, depending upon the length of the waiting lists at the hospital to which you have been sent . Having to go on to a long waiting list is one reason why some people decide to purchase a hearing aid privately. If you are told that there is a long waiting list, you could ask if there are any other centres at which you could be seen more quickly.

How do I buy an aid privately?

Anyone can go to a private hearing aid dispenser to purchase a hearing aid. The hearing aid dispenser is not compelled to suggest you seek medical advice, except for a certain number of prescribed conditions. These conditions are laid down by the Hearing Aid Council, which registers all private dispensers. But none the less it is advisable to obtain medical advice before getting a hearing aid for the first time. Wherever possible, it is better to purchase from a dispenser with a consulting room near to you than from someone who has to travel a long distance to see you at your home. In this way you are assured there is always an office to which you can return if you have problems with the aid.

If you decide to buy a hearing aid, no financial help will be given by the NHS; however, batteries for some types of privately purchased hearing aids are available through the NHS free of charge. Moreover, buying a private aid in no way prevents you from getting one through the NHS as well.

Due to the fact that hearing aids cannot be 'prescribed' in the same way as, say, spectacles, only the wearer can say if a hearing aid is giving sufficient benefit. When buying a hearing aid, it is important to have the aid on trial prior to completing the purchase. Many firms accept this as good practice and will permit trials on an agreed basis. If the company you go to first of all does not permit this, then perhaps you should try elsewhere. You should realise that you are paying mainly for this type of service, not just for the cost of the instrument itself.

If you buy a hearing aid privately, then you are given some protection by the Hearing Aid Council's Code of Practice, which must be followed by all hearing aid dispensers. Basically the code requires that dispensers should act in the best interests of the client and should not misrepresent themselves in any way; but perhaps the best protection of all, particularly for those who do choose to purchase a hearing aid at home, is to ask the dispenser to allow a free trial of any hearing aid supplied. If you decide to return the hearing aid within the trial period, then, provided that it is in good condition, any money you have paid should be returned. At the present time there are around three or four hundred dispensers in private practice; some work independently from their own consulting rooms, while others are employed by large national companies.

Hearing aid advertisements tend to over-simplify the problems of hearing impairment and often exaggerate the potential benefits a hearing aid may give, so their claims should be treated with caution.

How can I be sure that a hearing aid will help?

There is only one way to discover how much a hearing aid might help, and that is by trying one. Unlike glasses, the benefits may not be immediate and therefore it is important to try an aid over a period of time, while receiving help and guidance in its use. For some people it may take quite a while to adjust completely to using an aid, but within a couple of weeks any major problems should have become apparent. Further help can then be sought in overcoming them, perhaps by adjustment of the hearing aid or modification to the earmould.

In some NHS hearing aid clinics there will be a hearing therapist whose job involves helping people with their hearing problems after they have been given hearing aids. This can include providing help and advice on lip-reading and auditory training facilities (see Chapter 7).

How accurately can hearing aids be prescribed?

Because many people are familiar with the process of having glasses prescribed and fitted by an optician, they believe that hearing aids can be prescribed in the same way. An optician is able to make an accurate prescription for a lens that will correct simple optical imperfections of the eye; this prescription can be fulfilled by any competent lens manufacturer. But the situation is not nearly as straightforward when dealing with hearing loss; it is not possible, particularly when dealing with perceptive hearing loss, to produce a 'prescription' that will completely correct the hearing deficiency. The reason is that the defect in the ear lies in the mechanism that turns sound into 'neural' messages which go to the brain (a mechanism which is still not completely understood), so the problem is more like damage to the retina of the eye or the optic nerve, deficiencies which cannot be overcome by wearing glasses.

5 Hearing aids

How do they work?

Hearing aids come in a variety of shapes and sizes, some to be worn on the body, some behind the ear, and others within the bowl of the ear, or even within the ear canal itself. Hearing aids can also be built into or attached to spectacle frames. All these aids are amplifiers; they make sound louder. Although their appearance may vary, all aids have a similar set of functional parts, that is, microphone,

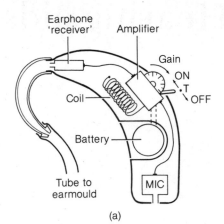

(a)

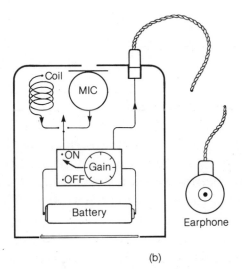

(b)

Fig. 4 Component parts of (a) a behind-the-ear and (b) a body worn hearing aid

amplifier with volume control, earphone and battery, and these are shown in Fig. 4. →There are, of course, differences between hearing aids apart from shape, such as in the range of tones which are amplified and the loudest sounds which can be delivered to the ear. It is very important to realise that the most suitable hearing aid for an individual is not neccessarily the most powerful, nor the one giving the highest level of amplification; moreover the one which is recommended by your best friend will not necessarily be the best for you.

What hearing aids are available?

Two types of hearing aids are available from the NHS: body-worn aids and those worn behind the ear (sometimes called post-aural) (see Fig. 5). A range of models to suit different hearing losses is available for each type. From the private sector, in-the-ear aids and aids built into spectacles (see Fig. 6) can be obtained in addition to body-worn and behind-the-ear aids, with several manufacturers providing a range of models in each type. Thus, according to the lists compiled by the Royal National Institute for the Deaf,

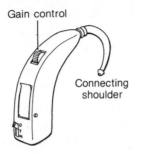

Gain control

Connecting
shoulder

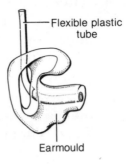

Flexible plastic
tube

Earmould

(a)

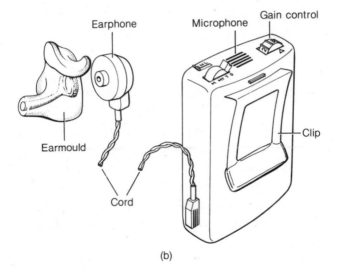

Earphone

Microphone

Gain control

Earmould

Cord

Clip

(b)

Fig. 5 National Health Service hearing aids: (a) a
behind-the-ear aid; (b) a typical body-worn aid

there are altogether some four hundred
models of hearing aids available in the
UK, of which rather more than half are of
the type worn behind the ear. It is
important to distinguish here between the
private hearing aid dispensers—the
people who actually sell hearing aids to the
public—and the manufacturers which are
often multinational electronics companies,

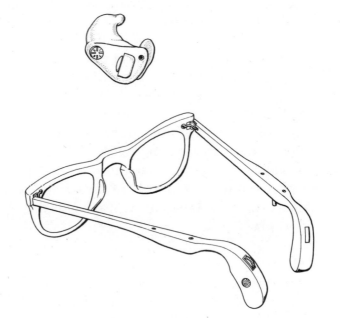

Fig. 6 (a) In-the-ear and (b) spectacle hearing aid

Most people will want a hearing aid to be inconspicuous, so body-worn hearing aids are now usually worn only by profoundly deaf people, or those whose finger and arm movements do not allow them to use the smaller aids. The other types of aids are often hardly noticeable when in place, especially if the wearer has hair which covers the ears.

What is an earmould?

An earmould is an important part of a complete hearing aid system; it is the part which connects the hearing aid to the ear (see Fig. 5). It is usually produced from an impression taken of the ear, in the same way that dentures are made. With body-worn aids, it conducts the sound from the earphone into the ear and, in the case of aids worn behind the ear, it also holds the aid in place.

If the earmould is not a good fit, it can cause discomfort and might cause the aid to whistle. This is known as 'feedback'. This whistle often is not heard by the wearer, but it can be annoying to other people and will limit the effectiveness of the hearing aid. Sometimes the earmould may have been poorly made, but often it turns out that the user has simply not fitted the mould correctly into the ear. This task is difficult for some people and the correct way has to be learned by practice. The particular choice of earmould can affect the amount and character of sound coming from the aid and the choice will generally be made by the dispenser or hearing aid technician.

Earmoulds become soiled with use and require changing from time to time. The plastic tubing which connects to hearing aids of the type worn behind the ear deteriorates with use and has to be replaced on a regular basis. Earmoulds are often charged for as an extra item when hearing aids are purchased privately. However, such earmoulds can usually be used with another hearing aid of similar type; so even if you are returning a hearing aid, the earmould should still be useful to you.

Can you adjust the tone of an aid?

Body-worn hearing aids normally have a

tone control that be adjusted by the user. The control may have the following markings — **H** for the emphasis of high

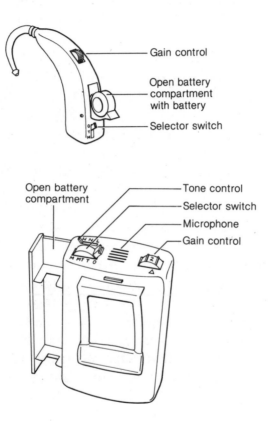

Gain control

Open battery compartment with battery

Selector switch

Open battery compartment

Tone control

Selector switch

Microphone

Gain control

Fig. 7 Hearing aid controls

tones, **N** for the normal response and **L** for the emphasis of low tones. The **H** position is useful for reducing the effects of any background noise when trying to listen to conversation. Figure 7 shows the controls that may be found on typical hearing aids. Due to their small size, head-worn aids often have no user-operated tone controls.

Besides the user's control, many hearing aids have small internal controls which can be pre-set by the supplier (using a jeweller's screwdriver) to give the sound that is likely to be of most benefit.

Do all hearing aids need a battery?

The only aids that do not require a battery are the acoustic aids such as ear trumpets and speaking tubes (see below). All other aids need some form of electrical power, usually provided by a replaceable battery. Rechargeable batteries are sometimes used and even solar cells, but the majority of batteries are of the type you discard after use.

Are ear trumpets still used?

The answer is, generally, no. However, the very small size of modern aids leads to obvious difficulties for those who do not have the physical or mental ability to handle small objects. Acoustic aids such as the ear trumpet or speaking tube have the advantage of larger size with no controls or batteries to manipulate. For people who are both elderly and frail these are

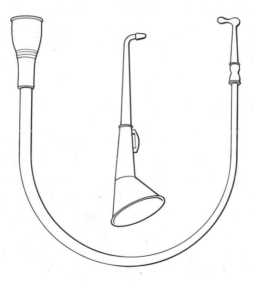

Fig. 8 Ear trumpet and speaking tube

sometimes the only means of amplification which are practical. The ear trumpet, and particularly the speaking tube, ought to be standard equipment in all residential homes and hospitals for the elderly and should be carried by all professionals working with such people, to allow for easier communication. The NHS still provides a small range of acoustic aids (see Fig. 8) and a few can be purchased privately.

Will my hearing get worse if I use an aid?

Many people think that once you start to use a hearing aid you will become dependent upon it and that your hearing will get worse. A hearing aid, if correctly selected, should not in itself cause your hearing to deteriorate, but it will not prevent your loss from becoming worse if it is of a progressive type. With the majority of people, however, changes in their hearing occur very slowly, and nearly everybody's hearing becomes less acute as they grow older. There is, therefore, no sense in delaying the use of a hearing aid and, consequently, foregoing the advantages it can bring.

Should I use an aid all the time?

When you first obtain a hearing aid, it is a good idea to use it for short periods of time in a fairly quiet place, such as your home. As you become used to it, you can try it out in various places outside your home, until you have the confidence to use it whenever it is needed.

Many people with small hearing losses require their aids only in certain circumstances; they do not need to wear them all the time. People with more severe losses may want to wear their aids all the time; they simply switch them off when not required.

Are there any situations in which a hearing aid is not helpful?

Most people who use hearing aids will tell you that they are most effective when they are used somewhere quiet, with only one person speaking, at a normal conversational distance. Once the person speaking moves away, or the place becomes noisy, the hearing aid becomes less effective. In fact, many people switch their aids off in very noisy surroundings as they feel they are better off without them.

These limitations of using hearing aids are unfortunate because a person with only a small loss of hearing may not need an aid for normal conversation, but may find it provides only limited benefit when the listening conditions are not so good, when help is really needed. Because the discovery of this fact can lead to dissatisfaction, it is important that potential hearing aid users are informed of these limitations and are properly counselled not to expect more help than a hearing aid can reasonably give. It is also important for people to know about other means of overcoming particular everyday problems, using various technical aids or devices—sometimes in conjunction with the hearing aid (see Chapter 6).

Do hearing aids really make speech clear?

This may seem a silly question to ask, as this is probably the reason why most people feel they need a hearing aid.

However, it must be remembered that sensorineural hearing loss reduces the ability to understand speech even when it is made sufficiently loud (see page 5). A hearing aid can help many people understand speech quite well, by making it louder, but by no means does this solve every problem. Therefore, just because someone uses an aid and is able to hear you speaking, it does not mean that the person can completely follow what you are saying; often that person will have to lip-read as well. Unfortunately, this can lead to misunderstandings when people are talking to hearing aid users; sometimes there is a tendency to think, quite wrongly, that they are being stupid or difficult. The hearing aid will make good the loss of sound intensity, but it will not restore the loss of discrimination in the ear itself.

Are two aids better than one?

In theory, two hearing aids should be better as they provide natural binaural hearing (two-eared listening), but in practice a single aid is often preferred as it is more easily managed. If the hearing loss in one ear is much greater than in the other, the poorer ear might give distorted sound and only make things more difficult if a hearing aid is fitted to that ear. However, if two aids can be used successfully, they should be fitted, because it might then be easier to hear reasonably well in a noisy place or to tell from which direction a sound is coming. Through the NHS two hearing aids can be issued for simultaneous use if recommended by a consultant, but spare aids are only available to people with additional handicaps.

What is the 'T' switch position for?

When you switch your hearing aid to 'T' the microphone is disconnected and in its place a pick-up coil comes into use (see Fig. 4). This tiny coil of wire picks up 'magnetic waves' from a 'loop system' (see page 70) or a telephone 'inductive coupler' (see page 73). You should find that background noise is minimised and speech may be clearer when one of these facilities has been installed. This can be of help when you are using the telephone, television, or when you are in church or other public places where a loop system is fitted.

The following sign (Fig. 9) perhaps with a 'T' printed on it may indicate that a loop facility is provided.

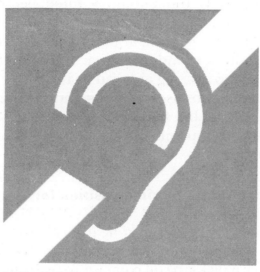

Fig. 9 World Federation of the Deaf symbol

What sort of hearing aids are used by children?

Children use the same type of personal hearing aids as adults; hearing aids are not designed specifically for children.
However, children's hearing aids are often used in conjunction with other equipment, in particular radio receivers.

Present-day policy in the education of hearing-impaired children is to enable as many children as possible to go to the same schools as normally hearing children. Where this is not possible, a Partially Hearing Unit (PHU) attached to a normal school may cater for the child's needs. In the PHU a specially qualified teacher of the deaf will see to the special needs of the child,while as many lessons as possible will be taken in normal classes with the other children. Those children who cannot manage in a PHU will go to a special school for the deaf, which will usually only take children with severe or profound hearing losses. No matter which type of schooling the child is given, the problems of listening in a noisy classroom, or at a distance from the teacher, will still be present (see page 52). However, these problems can be alleviated by using either the loop system (see page 70) or sets of wearable radio microphone aids.

Radio aids consist of two parts. The teacher wears a radio transmitter coupled to a microphone, which may be built in or attached to a lead so that it can be fixed to the clothing, such as a jacket lapel. The transmitter is very similar to the type

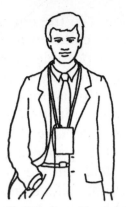

Fig. 10 Radio microphone transmitter

which you may have seen being worn by television presenters so that they do not have to talk into a fixed microphone. The signals from the transmitter are picked up by radio receivers worn by the children. The receiver may be part of a special hearing aid (Fig. 11a) or a separate unit which can be connected to an ordinary hearing aid. The connection is often by means of a small induction loop (see Fig. 11b), which is worn around the neck (with the hearing aid set to **T**), but sometimes the link is by a direct wire (Fig. 11c) if the hearing aid has a socket fitted for this purpose. There is no technical reason why these systems cannot be used by adults, but their main use is in education.

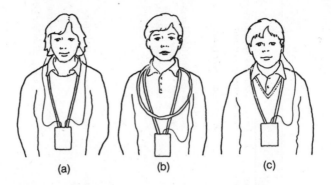

Fig. 11 Three ways to receive "sound": (a) Combined radio receiver and hearing aid; (b) Radio receiver connected to induction loop and behind-the-ear hearing aid switched to T; and (c) Radio receiver directly connected to behind-the-ear aid

How can you test a hearing aid?

The chart on the next two pages lists the faults most likely to occur in body-worn and behind-the-ear aids together with some simple checks which will show whether a hearing aid is working correctly or not. A full technical test can only be undertaken using special electronic equipment and this should be carried out by the supplier after any repairs have been done.

Finding faults in your hearing aid.
(a) Body worn aids

Symptoms	Items to check	Fault	Action
Aid dead	Earmould	Earmould blocked with wax	Unclip from receiver and clean.
	Battery	Battery flat. Wrong way round.	Examine/replace. Insert correctly.
		Contacts dirty or broken	
	Cord	Cord broken or intermittent	Wiggle cord near plugs. Replace.
	Receiver	Faulty receiver or socket	Replace.
	Body of Aid	Faulty socket	Move cord in and out of socket. Return aid for repair.
Rushing noise from aid	'T' switch	Switch in loop position or microphone not working	Switch to 'M' position. Return aid for repair.
Low output from aid	Battery, receiver, switch positions	Battery flat	
		Faulty or wrong receiver	
		Wrong setting of output/tone control	
Crackling	Cord, cord plug socket volume control	Intermittent cord, dirty volume control	Replace cord, clean volume control. Repair aid.
		Faulty socket	
Acoustic feedback	Earmould	Poor fitting earmould	Check fit of earmould. Replace.
Electrical feedback	Battery contacts	Low voltage causing electrical instability	Change battery; clean contact.

(b) Behind-the-ear aids

Symptoms	Items to check	Fault	Action
Aid dead	Earmould	Earmould blocked with wax/moisture	Remove earmould and clear.
	Battery	Battery flat, wrong way round, dirty contacts	Examine, test/replace. Insert correctly.
Rushing noise	'T' switch	Switch in loop position. Microphone not working	Reset switch to 'M' position. Return aid for repair.
Low output	Setting of output/tone control	Reset controls	Return aid for repair.
	Earmould and tubing	Blockage	Remove blockage.
Crackling	Battery contacts, switches, volume control	Faulty connections	Clean contacts if possible. Return for repair.
Acoustic feedback	Earmould, tubing connecting shoulder	Split in tube or leakage of some kind	Replace tube, etc.
Mechanical feedback	Aid produces whistling noise when sound outlet is blocked off	Possible poor mounting of microphone or earphone	Return for repair.

What are cochlear implants?

Cochlear implants are not transplants. In a transplant operation an organ is removed from the body of one person and placed into another body. An implant, however, is an artificial device imbedded into the body which, through electrical stimulation of appropriate nerve endings, allows the body to function, when previously it could not do so in the normal way.

Cochlear implants involve the surgical implantation of an electrode, which is designed to carry a tiny electrical current into or on to the cochlea (inner ear). The currents for this electrode are provided by a box of sophisticated electronics which processes the sound picked up by a microphone. The complete unit can then be used as a type of hearing aid. To improve the appearance of the device and minimise the risk of infection, no direct connection is normally made between the implanted electrode and the external processor box. The currents for the electrode are induced remotely into a special coil, which is implanted under the skin close to the ear, from a similar coil held in place behind the ear (see Fig. 12).

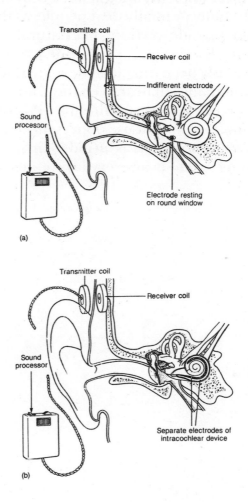

Fig. 12 Cochlear implants: (a) Single channel implant with electrode resting on the round window; (b) Multi-channel implant with electrode inside cochlea

Cochlear implants are intended only for profoundly or totally deaf people, as they do not provide anything like natural hearing. However, for someone who has previously been unable to hear anything at all, the chance to hear even the crudest of sounds can be very worth while. Probably the most important use of present-day cochlear implants is as an aid to lip-reading and to hear everyday sounds.

6 Are there any other aids?

What are aids to daily living?

We have explained how hearing aids can assist with many problems caused by impaired hearing, but have stressed that their uses are limited. There are situations in which hearing aids will not help; for instance, very few people wear them in bed and therefore cannot hear an ordinary alarm clock. Many people cannot hear the doorbell, particularly if they do not wear their hearing aid at home, and listening to television is not always satisfactory with a hearing aid. There are, however, devices which will often be more useful than a personal hearing aid in these situations; some of these are described in this chapter. Such aids are sometimes known as environmental aids or assistive devices. We have called them aids to daily living.

How can I hear someone at the door?

This is a common problem, especially if you live alone. A bell with a different tone might help and you could put extension bells in the rooms you use most often. Local stores often have attractive displays of bells, buzzers and chimes for you to try.

If you cannot hear any of these sounds there are special 'doorbells' with flashing lights to attract your attention. The most widely known type works by flashing the ordinary lights in the room you are in when someone presses the bell, but there are other systems which are available to suit different requirements. Some of these are portable, with their own built-in lights powered by batteries; others must be plugged into the mains, but are still designed to be installed yourself. However, most of the systems which run from the electric mains, particularly the type which flashes the ordinary house lights, must be installed by an electrician.

A dog can act as a useful pair of ears, telling you when someone is at the door. A few people have specially trained 'hearing dogs' to help them to respond to various sounds around the home.

Can I get a special alarm clock?

If you cannot hear your alarm, it is difficult to get up on time. Conventional clockwork alarms and modern electronic alarms produce different kinds of sounds, so it is worth trying a few models to see if you can find one that suits you. If you cannot find one that will wake you, you can get special alarms that will. These work by either flashing a light at your bedside or by vibrating a special pad placed under your mattress or pillow.

How can I hear my baby cry?

It can be very worrying if your hearing loss prevents you from hearing when your baby cries. There is, however, a simple device to help with this problem—a baby alarm which uses a flashing light instead of sound to attract your attention. The light flashes in time with the baby's cries, so you can tell how much the baby is crying. You can obtain a version of the alarm with a vibrator pad (to place under your mattress) if you find the flashing light ineffective while you are sleeping.

Baby alarms are sometimes known as 'visual indicators', because these units can be used around the house whenever you need to convert a warning sound in to a flashing light or vibration.

How can I hear the television without disturbing my neighbours?

Surveys have shown that listening to television is the problem most often mentioned by people with hearing difficulties. Friction with the family and neighbours, when the person tries to raise the volume, is often the reason for the person eventually seeking help.

There is no need to endure this frustration, because on many TV sets sockets are fitted into which you can plug headphones or a special TV listening aid. You should find out whether doing this cuts off the loudspeaker in the set, if others in the room want to listen as well. Your TV dealer should be able to advise you on this, and also on the choice of suitable headphones.

If your hearing loss is more severe, you may be better off with a special listening aid. Some of these can be plugged into the set, while others pick up the sound by a small microphone fixed near the loudspeaker in the set. This is quite useful if the TV set does not have an earphone socket. You could also have an induction loop fitted (see next section), so that you can listen through your own hearing aid, set to 'T'.

What is the 'loop system'?

An induction loop is a system which is used in conjunction with a hearing aid having a switch with a position marked 'T' (see page 55). The loop works on the simple principle that when an electric current passes through a wire it produces a magnetic field around that wire. If the wire is then formed into a loop, a magnetic field is produced throughout the area enclosed by the loop. The loop itself could be big enough to cover completely the interior of a cathedral or small enough to go into a telephone earpiece; provided there is an adequate level of current flowing in the wire, a satisfactory level of magnetic field will be provided. The magnetic field can be picked up by a small coil of wire (rather like an aerial) built into the hearing aid. The coil is selected by moving the switch to the position marked 'T' on the hearing aid and the aid then converts the magnetic field back in to sound for the listener to hear. If the current flowing through the loop wire comes from an amplifier, which in turn obtains its signal from, say, a TV set, the listener will hear the sound as if it were coming directly from the set's loudspeaker—but without the distraction of other sounds, such as people talking, and without any echoes from the room itself (see Fig. 13).

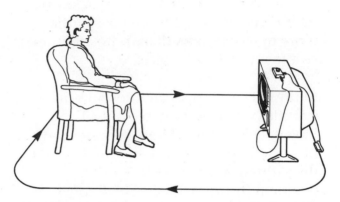

Fig. 13 Loop system for listening to the television

What is Teletext?

Both the BBC and the IBA transmit large electronic 'magazines' of information through the Teletext system. The information appears on your TV screen in the form of text and simple diagrams, provided you have a Teletext TV set (you can buy an add-on 'decorder' if you do not possess a Teletext set). The BBC's service is called Ceefax and the IBA's is called Oracle. Both have special 'magazines' for people with hearing problems, 'No Need to Shout' on Ceefax and 'Earshot' on Oracle. You select the page you want to look at from your remote control key pad. Although Teletext TV sets cost a little more to rent or buy, there is no additional cost to receive the service.

Many television programmes now have subtitles which you can see only if you have a Teletext set. These subtitles can be of great help if you have hearing difficulties. As a free service the Royal National Institute for the Deaf, together with the BBC, provides synopses of certain forthcoming plays and drama series. If these are read beforehand the action can be followed more easily.

What about the telephone?

There are two problems you may have with the telephone. You may not be able to hear when it rings and/or you may not be able to hear what the person is saying once you have answered.

If you cannot hear when the telephone rings, you can buy a flashing light system and have it connected to your telephone by British Telecom. Portable systems are available which require no internal connection to the telephone. If you work in an office, a telephone with a small flashing lamp built in may help. It would even be possible to be woken at night by a vibrator unit attached to the telephone.

If your hearing loss is not very serious, you may find that you can still use the telephone without further help. But if your hearing loss is more severe, you can get an 'amplified handset' with a volume control, or an 'inductive coupler' (a miniature induction loop) fitted into the telephone earpiece with which you use your hearing aid switched to 'T'. Public telephones equipped with this facility are marked with the international symbol indicating help for hearing-impaired people (see Fig. 9).

Even if you are profoundly deaf, an extra earpiece on the telephone, called a 'watch receiver', will allow a hearing person to listen in. You can then lip-read this person repeating the words for you.

How can the telephone be used by a person with no hearing?

One possible solution would be to use a video telephone system which allowed each party to see the other and therefore to lip-read or communicate normally. Unfortunately, although such systems exist, they cannot yet be used on the public telephone network. However, modern electronics have made it possible for totally deaf people to use the telephone by means of special keyboard terminals. The important point to remember with this type of equipment is that a terminal is required by both parties and that the terminals have to be compatible with each other. Not all terminals can 'talk' to each other in this way, but some popular personal computers, for example, can be made to do this using appropriate adaptors (known as 'modems').

Efforts are being made to agree a standard to which all systems that might be used by deaf people should conform; this would ensure that your machine would be able to communicate with someone else's machine of a different make.

At the moment there is only one terminal which has been made specifically for deaf people; it is battery operated and acoustically coupled to the telephone. That means you simply place the telephone handset into a pair of rubber cups on the machine, and pulses of sound are sent into the telephone mouthpiece from one machine and received by the other machine through the telephone earpiece. The machine is relatively expensive, especially bearing in mind that two are required to carry out a conversation.

A more general approach is to use a 'viewdata' adaptor. A viewdata adaptor connected to your telephone line allows you to receive information over the telephone and this can be viewed on a TV screen. These adaptors are mains operated, but suitable for any fixed position at home or at work. The system is most commonly used to receive a wide range of general information (news, weather reports, etc.) through services such as British Telecom's Prestel, but the electronic 'Mailbox' facility, which allows one subscriber to leave messages for another subscriber, is of special interest to deaf people. The messages are typed on the keyboard of your viewdata adaptor and are stored in electronic 'pigeon holes' until they are read by the recipient. Special codes can be entered from your keyboard so that no one else can read the messages which have been left for you.

How can a deaf person speak to a person with no special equipment over the telephone?

Although electronic terminals allow a deaf person to 'talk' to another person with a suitable terminal, the majority of normally hearing people will not have this special equipment. A Telephone Exchange for the deaf has been introduced by the Royal National Institute for the Deaf to help overcome this problem. The exchange, which operates only from Central London at the moment, allows a deaf person with a viewdata terminal to communicate with a hearing person (who does not have the special equipment), through an operator. The operator listens to what the hearing person is saying and types it so that it appears on the deaf person's screen. Figure 14 shows how the system works.

Many people believe that it is possible for computers to turn speech into the printed form. Unfortunately, although major advances have been made in this area, and some computers can be 'trained' to respond to a limited number of commands from a particular voice, no computer is

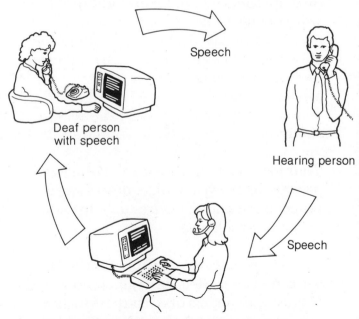

Fig. 14 The telephone exchange for the deaf

able to transcribe ordinary conversation into print.

Where can I buy these aids?

Unfortunately it is not always easy to buy some of the aids which have been described. Many are produced by small companies, so purchase by mail order is common. They cannot be obtained through the NHS, but your local social services may provide financial help towards purchase and/or installation. It is always worth getting in touch with them to find out their policy. The level of assistance varies from one borough to another, so it is not possible to generalise about the help available in your area.

Your local area telephone sales office can provide you with a booklet describing a range of telephone devices to help with different problems.

The Royal National Institute for the Deaf will send you leaflets describing most types of aids, with details of what they do, how much they cost and where to get hold of them.

7 What else can I do?

Can I learn to lip-read?

You can attend lip-reading classes in many parts of the country, where specialist teachers of lip-reading provide tuition. We all lip-read to some extent; this is why we find it annoying when the sound is not properly synchronised to the vision on films and TV. Therefore many people find they can lip-read quite well if they have to. At classes you can learn how to place yourself in the best position to lip-read, and how to use the various clues to understand what is being said. Even the best lip-reader probably only reads 50 per cent of words on the lips; the rest must be guessed from the context of what is being said.

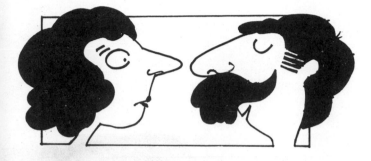

Classes can also be very good places to socialise and they allow people with hearing problems to learn from the experiences of others.

What is auditory training?

The main purpose of auditory training is to teach you to make the best use of the (distorted) sounds you may hear if you have a severe perceptive hearing loss. Amplification is provided by means of a personal hearing aid or a desk model auditory training unit. Auditory training sessions are often run in conjunction with lip-reading classes.

How can other people help?

Our ability to communicate is strongly influenced by what other people do. In particular, lip-reading is impossible if the speaker stands against the light, or in shadow, or speaks with a cigarette in his or her mouth. It can be very difficult to follow a conversation if you are not familiar with the subject, or if the speaker suddenly switches to a different topic.

It helps a great deal if other people understand the deaf person's problems. They should realise that communication may be difficult and that sometimes things have to be written down or repeated. Perhaps the most difficult thing for deaf people to comprehend is that other people may feel irritated by their deafness. This is not a pleasant fact, but it should, at least, be understood.

You should face a deaf person directly when speaking; speak slightly more slowly than usual, but do not shout. Shouting distorts the facial features and does not help at all. Above all, speak clearly; people with hearing loss often complain that others are mumbling—and quite often it is true.

Can I register as a disabled person?

Depending upon your degree of hearing loss, you may be able to register as disabled. The social services department of your local authority will tell you how to go about this. If you register as disabled, it may not, however, prove very helpful, as there are very few benefits to be obtained.

8 Who else can I turn to for help?

Which government bodies can help?

The social services department of your local authority is the first official body you might approach for help, because under the terms of the Chronically Sick and Disabled Persons Act they have an obligation to help people who have problems in coping with hearing loss. Some authorities employ specialist Social Workers with the Deaf, trained to deal with the problems of people born deaf and the hard of hearing: you should ask to speak to this person. Social services are permitted to pay for technical aids, and depending on the policy of your local authority, may provide TV listening aids, special doorbells, etc. You should check with your social services department, who can be found through your local council.

At your local Job Centre a Disablement Resettlement Officer can advise on, and try to find work for a disabled person. Hearing loss is a disability which often makes finding a job more difficult. The Manpower Services Commission (MSC) funds training courses for disabled people and can provide aids to help people in work. The Job Centre can tell you how to contact the MSC.

Hearing Aid Council
40a Ludgate Hill
London, EC4M 7DE

The Hearing Aid Council was set up by an Act of Parliament to register private dispensers of hearing aids. The council issues a code of practice and can discipline dispensers who break this code. If you have recently purchased a hearing aid and feel that you have a grievance, you can refer your complaint to the Hearing Aid Council. It is not, however, an advice-giving body on hearing aids and deafness.

Are there any voluntary organisations?

There are many hundreds of organisations which have been set up to help hearing-impaired people in various ways. In your own area you may find several organisations, each dealing with a different aspect of hearing loss. However, the four main national organisations come together as the 'Panel of Four' in order to meet officially with the Minister for the Disabled. These organisations are the Royal National Institute for the Deaf, the British Association of the Hard of Hearing, the National Deaf Children's Society and the British Deaf Association.

The Royal National Institute for the Deaf (RNID)
105 Gower Street
London WCIE 6AH
(Tel: 01-387 8033)

This organisation offers help to people of

all ages and with any degree of hearing loss. It provides residential accommodation and training for profoundly deaf people and supports scientific and medical research. It runs a free Hearing Advisory Service staffed by professional workers, which specialises in the problems associated with hearing impairment. The organisation also includes the British Tinnitus Association, which was formed by RNID to advise people suffering from tinnitus. It has helped to establish self-help groups around the country.

British Association of the Hard of Hearing (BAHOH)
7–11 Armstrong Road
London W3 7JL
(Tel: 01-743 1110)

This body organises clubs for hard of hearing people throughout the country. The clubs provide meeting places for adults with all degrees of hearing loss. Lip-reading classes are run by some clubs.

National Deaf Children's Society (NDCS)
45 Hereford Road
London W2
(Tel: 01-229 9272/4)

This society organises local groups for parents of deaf children throughout the country. It provides advice, particularly on educational and welfare matters concerning children.

British Deaf Association (BDA)
38 Victoria Place
Carlisle
(Tel: 0228-48844)

This organisation is mainly concerned with people who communicate by sign language and finger spelling. It provides specialist services and organises clubs for profoundly deaf people.

What about clubs and societies?

Local clubs and societies for the hearing-imparied vary in size and range of activities. Some deal only with deaf people who use sign language, but many cater for hard-of-hearing people. Your Citizens' Advice Bureau, social services department or notice board of your local library will tell you if there is a club or society in your area. Alternatively, you could write to either BDA or BAHOH.

Appendix 1
Glossary

Air conduction

A term usually associated with audiometry
and referring to sound being heard
through earphones.

Amplified handset

A telephone handset with a built-in
amplifier.

Audiogram

A chart showing the degree of hearing loss in decibels over a range of tones (frequencies).

Audiometer

An electronic instrument used for measuring the threshold of hearing.

Audiometry

The procedures by which the threshold of hearing is measured.

Auditory training unit

A desk-top hearing aid often used in the education of deaf children.

Auricle

The visible part of the ear. Also known as the pinna.

Binaural

Listening with both ears.

Body-worn aid

A hearing aid in which the microphone, amplifier and battery are housed in a small unit worn on the body. The earphone is connected by a lead (cord) to the aid.

Bone conduction

The process by which sound is heard from a vibrator placed on the skull, usually behind the ear.

Bone vibrator

A vibrator used for bone conduction audiometry, or with certain types of hearing aids.

Conductive hearing loss

A hearing loss associated with the functioning of the outer or middle ear.

Deaf

The *Concise Oxford English Dictionary* gives the following definition: 'wholly or partly without hearing'.

Decibel (dB)

A unit of measurement widely used in the fields of sound, hearing, radio, etc. Often followed by other letters which give extra information about the type of measurement being made, for example, dB(A) is a measurement made with a sound level meter on its 'A weighting network'; this takes less account of low tones to give better agreement with how people will hear the loudness of sound.

Earmould

A piece of plastic, usually moulded to the shape of an individual's ear, that conducts sound from the hearing aid into the ear.

Earphone (receiver)

The part of the hearing aid (or separate device) that produces the sound.

ENT clinic

Short for ear, nose and throat clinic, where hearing loss is diagnosed and treated.

Feedback

Acoustic feedback, oscillation, whistling, are terms that are used to describe what happens when too much amplified sound 'escapes' from the ear and is picked up by the microphone of the hearing aid. The result can be heard as high-pitched whistling. The whistling will persist until the amplification of the hearing aid is reduced (that is, the gain control is turned down).

Frequency

The number of sound vibrations per second, expressed as Hertz (Hz). This corresponds to the pitch of sound; high frequency means high pitch and vice versa.

Hard of hearing

A term normally used to describe someone who uses or might use a hearing aid.

Head-worn aid

A hearing aid worn entirely on the head, either behind the ear, in the bowl of the ear, in a spectacle arm or on a headband.

Hearing loss

The difference between the level of sound that can just be heard by an individual with impaired hearing and a standard level which has been found by averaging measurements from a group of young normally hearing people (usually expressed in decibels).

Induction loop

An induction loop is often in the form of a wire, run around the perimeter of a room, which is fed by an audio amplifier with an electric current. This current produces a magnetic field which can then be picked up by a coil of wire in the hearing aid (selected by moving the switch to 'T') and heard as sound by the user.

Inductive coupler

A coil of wire which acts like a miniature induction loop system that is fitted in, or attached to, a telephone earphone to allow a hearing aid user to hear more easily on the telephone. The aid must have a 'T' switch position.

Inner ear

That part of the ear (mainly the cochlea) that converts mechanical vibrations (sound) into 'neural messages' that are sent to the brain.

Lip-reading (speech-reading)

The ability to understand what is being said by watching the lips. Usually involves watching the whole face and neck as well.

Loudness discomfort level

The level of sound which the listener finds uncomfortable to listen to for any length of time.

Masker

A device, usually worn behind the ear, that produces a rushing noise which may help reduce (mask) internal head noises (tinnitus).

Masking

The process by which the audibility of one sound is reduced by the presence of another sound.

Middle ear

That part of the ear which conducts sound to the inner ear. It consists of the eardrum, middle ear bones (ossicles) and the cavity containing them.

Otosclerosis

A condition in which the bones of the middle ear become covered with a bony growth.

Ototoxic

Applied to drugs that can damage hearing.

Perceptive hearing loss

See sensorineural hearing loss.

Pick-up coil

A small coil of many turns of fine wire, used in hearing aids to pick up the magnetic field from a loop system.

Post-aural (auricular)

Commonly used name to describe hearing aids worn behind the ear.

Pre-lingually

Deafness occuring before speech and language has developed normally in a child.

Presbyacusis

Hearing loss associated with elderly people.

Pure tone

A continuous sound occuring at one frequency only. Used in audiometry.

Receiver

See earphone.

Sensorineural hearing loss

A hearing loss that occurs in the inner ear or pathways to the brain, causing distortion of sounds and making speech difficult to understand. Not usually possible to alleviate by surgical or medical means.

Semicircular canals

The organ of balance which is connected directly to the cochlea.

Speech audiometry

The testing of hearing with speech, usually lists of isolated words but possibly sentences, etc.

Speech trainer

See auditory training unit.

Teletext

A system which allows printed and graphical information to be transmitted on TV channels which can be viewed on a TV set.

Temporary threshold shift (TTS)

A loss of hearing which disappears after a period of recovery. Often associated with the effect of loud noise.

Threshold of hearing

The faintest sound that can be consistently heard in an audiometric test.

Tinnitus

Noises in the head or ears.

Vestibular function

The body's control of balance by the ears, eyes and brain.

Watch receiver

A separate additional earphone attached to the telephone. Usually used by a normally hearing person so that what is being said can be relayed to a deaf person who replies into the telephone.

Appendix 2 Professional people who work with hearing-impaired people

Audiological scientist

A scientist who is usually hospital-based and is concerned with the identification and diagnosis of hearing impairment as well as the rehabilitation of hearing-impaired patients, both children and adults.

Hearing aid practitioner (dispenser)

Hearing aid practitioners prescribe and dispense hearing aids in the private sector in accordance with the Hearing Aid Council Act (1968). They carry out sufficient audiometric testing, auroscope examination and case-history investigation to enable appropriate provision of a hearing aid. The dispenser will select, adjust and fit hearing aids, specifying and preparing appropriate earmoulds and carrying out any necessary acoustic modification of the ear-fitting. They will instruct in the use of hearing aids, give rehabilitative advice, and re-assess at intervals, with consequent adjustments or changes.

Hearing therapist

After a hearing aid has been issued by the hospital, the hearing therapist assesses the rehabilitative needs of those suffering with acquired deafness, provides help with communication using hearing aids and environmental aids, and teaches the skills of speech-reading and auditory training.

Industrial audiometrist

Industrial audiometrists undertake

evaluation of the pure tone thresholds of hearing of persons working in industry, and they are responsible for the categorisation of the results. The work undertaken by an industrial audiometrist may also include selection and provision of hearing protectors, the education of workers, noise measurement and various aspects of noise control.

Lip-reading teacher

The lip-reading teacher undertakes the teaching of lip-reading to post-lingually deafened adults (sixteen years and over). This is usually class teaching to groups of around ten students, as communication with the group is seen as a valuable part of the work, but individual teaching may be offered where necessary or desirable.

Otolaryngologist

A surgeon who specialises in the diagnosis and medical, surgical and rehabilitational management of disorders, diseases and injuries of the ear, nose and throat.

Teacher of the deaf

A qualified teacher who has undertaken additional compulsory training leading to a qualification to teach children with impaired hearing. He or she is employed in special schools, units associated with normal schools, peripatetic services, hospitals, etc. Such teachers act in an advisory capacity to local education authorities, parents and others according to the conditions of their appointments.

Teacher of the deaf (audiology) (educational audiologist)

A teacher of the deaf who has undertaken additional approved training in audiology leading to a recognised qualification. He or she is employed in special schools, educational and health services, and has specialist expertise in ascertaining and assessing losses of hearing in children, in recommending hearing aids, and giving guidance to parents on audiological matters and advising authorities accordingly.

The above descriptions have been
extracted from the British Society of
Audiology booklet, *Careers in Audiology*
which is available for £1 from:
British Society of Audiology
Harvest House
62 London Road
Reading
Berkshire RG15AS.

Otologist

This is an ear, nose and throat surgeon who specialises in problems of the ear.

Physician in audiological medicine

A consultant physician who has specialised in disorders of hearing and balance. This includes the investigation, diagnosis, medical and rehabilitative treatment of patients with such disorders. This is a relatively new profession with about twenty physicians currently practising.

Physiological measurement technician (audiology)

Audiology technicians routinely measure and evaluate the hearing capacity of adults and children, prepare individually moulded ear inserts, fit hearing aids, give training and guidance to patients in the use of hearing aids, and make minor repairs and adjustments where necessary.

Social worker with the deaf

A social worker with the deaf is usually employed in a local authority social work department to help hearing-impaired people cope with the social, environmental and personal difficulties that sometimes accompany their disability. He or she also offers support to families of people with such handicaps. A social worker with the deaf assesses the client's overall social work and service needs, mobilises and co-ordinates appropriate services and resources and acts as a consultant to colleagues.

Speech therapist

A speech therapist is concerned with the assessment and treatment of all types of communication disorders in children and adults. Problems include disorders of articulation, language (in which both understanding of the spoken and written word may be impaired), voice and fluency.